JAN MELARA

Vitrectomy With Face-Down Recovery: A Nurse's Journey

First edition

This book was professionally typeset on Reedsy.
Find out more at reedsy.com

Contents

Foreword

I'm an RN. I worked in an operating room for over twenty-five years and saw all manner of gruesome sights. But eye surgery still grosses me out.

Throughout my career as a surgical nurse, I would do anything to avoid ophthalmic (eye) cases. Neuro (brain), orthopedic (bone), cardiac (heart) surgery—I was fine with them all except ophthalmic (eye) surgery. No eyeballs for me! It was as if a giant picture of an eye with a great big slash drawn through it hung somewhere deep within my brain.

So, in September of 2014, I was pretty upset to find that I needed a trans pars plana vitrectomy. Just the thought of surgical instruments entering my eye was terrifying. Then, I discovered I would need to be face-down for at least a week after undergoing surgery. The combination was an emotional double whammy that just about knocked me to my knees.

But, the alternative was central blindness in my right eye. I chose surgery and the subsequent face-down recovery.

What follows is an account of my personal journey through vitrectomy and face-down recovery. If readers can pick up any helpful hints or tips, then my purpose in writing this book will be served. ***However, each eye is different, each surgeon is different, and each surgery is a case unto itself: follow your own doctor's orders to the letter and always let your personal physician's advice trump anything you read in this book.***

Let us begin.

I

My Vitrectomy

1

Houston, we have a problem.

It was early spring in the Carolinas and I sat on my back porch enjoying our much-prized lake view. I turned my head at the soft fluttering of a dove's wings as it landed in the flowerbed to my right. While trying to see the bird, I noticed that one section of the porch railing seemed strangely crooked. Almost an s-shape, in fact.

Odd, I thought, *must be those cheap internet glasses I bought.* Except that I'd been wearing those same glasses for over a year and the railing had never looked distorted before. I told myself it must be some residual deficit from a laser repair of my left retina years earlier. That explanation worked fine until I determined that the distortion was only visible through my right eye.

Heart pounding, I headed to the computer to Google "visual distortion wavy lines." A ton of information was delivered to my screen, none of it very reassuring.

It was time to quit horsing around. After telling my husband, Gary, about the change in my vision, I made an appointment with our local ophthalmology practice.

Then I waited. And tried in vain not to worry.

* * *

Finally, the afternoon of the appointment rolled around. Even in the ophthalmologist's waiting room, I kept closing my left eye and looking at straight objects with my right eye, hoping the distortion would be gone. It wasn't.

A tech led me though a battery of exams and tests, none of which were painful or really even uncomfortable. The simplest, an eye-chart vision test, was emotionally uncomfortable, though. It showed that the vision in my right eye was terrible, even with my glasses on.

Next came my time with the ophthalmologist himself. He did a slit-lamp exam just like in all the eye visits I'd ever had. Except this time, instead of handing me a prescription for new eyeglasses, he told me I had something called vitreomacular traction. It was serious and could lead to blindness. He wanted me to see a retinologist in Greenville, the nearest city large enough to have such a specialized practice. "The retinologist will do one of three things," my doctor said, holding up the corresponding number of fingers. "He'll watch it, give you a series of injections, or recommend surgery." I prayed for the first option as the receptionist made an appointment for me with the retinologist.

Then I waited a couple of weeks. During that time, I learned as much as I could about vitreomacular traction. It wasn't good. From what I could tell, if it was bad enough to cause distorted vision, then it wasn't going to resolve on its own. So, the waiting option seemed non-viable. Also, the injections my doctor had mentioned as option two were *intra-ocular* injections. I cringed at the thought of someone coming at my poor eye with a needle. And the final option, surgery, was just too gruesome to even contemplate. I took a little glance at the procedure anyway and to me it looked like endoscopy for the eye. Not as bad as it might be, but bad enough. I started waking up in the middle of the night worrying about what the retinologist would have to say once he examined my eye.

* * *

The retinologist's office was large, with three spacious waiting rooms. It needed to be big to accommodate a practice with so many doctors on staff. This bigness reassured me. To me, having multiple doctors working together meant that none of them would be taking call too frequently. Hence, whoever was on call would be fresh and rested, just the way I wanted someone who might be dealing with any eye emergency I might have. Also, I felt a large group would likely have policies and procedures in place to insure a high level of care.

Still, I was almost trembling as I went through the dilation, testing, and slit-lamp exam in the reassuringly large office. No matter how skilled these guys were, there was still something bad wrong with my eye and that scared the bejesus out of me.

Finally, we reached the part of the visit where the retinologist revealed the results of all the light-flashing and picture-taking. I had just what the ophthalmologist back in little old Laurens had said I had: vitreomacular traction. It was in such an early stage, though, that there was a fifty percent chance it would just resolve on its own. I brought up what I'd learned in my internet search—that once the thing was bad enough to cause symptoms, it was not likely to go away without some help. My doctor said the visual distortion I was experiencing was minor. I agreed. I couldn't even tell I had a problem unless I closed one eye and looked at a straight object just right. Heck, I was still able to thread needles with no problem. We decided to wait and watch. I was to return in six weeks.

It was the outcome I'd wished for, and yet I had a sick feeling this was not something that would disappear on its own. I spent a lot of time closing one eye and looking at the window blinds in my dining room, hoping the slats would appear as straight as they actually were. Instead, though, those slats kept getting more and more crooked when viewed through my right eye. I began to think of my right eye as my "bad" eye.

* * *

Gary drove me to my second appointment with the retinologist and we both dreaded what he would say, although I had convinced myself that my eyesight was somewhat improved. Certainly it was no worse.

The results of the eye-chart vision test showed differently. My vision had declined quite a bit in the six weeks since my original visit. The OCT (Ocular Coherence Tomography) told an equally dismal tale. The vitreous was pulling the retina like a band-aid tugging on skin. Even my untrained eye could see that something had to give.

We discussed the eye injections. Just talking about them made me a little nauseous. Luckily, my doctor didn't really think they were right for me. Of course, the alternative treatment was vitrectomy, an even more terrifying option. I quailed at the thought of three tubes—however tiny—being inserted into my poor baby eye and the vitreous being sucked out through one of them.

"I don't think I can do the face-down recovery because I have allergies. My nose would get stuffed up if I stayed face down for that long," I told the retinologist in an attempt to stave off surgery.

I could take decongestants if that happened, he countered.

"But a lot of those decongestants raise intraocular pressure! You wouldn't want that after surgery, would you?"

6

He smiled. "It would be fine. Not a problem."

Dang. Failed on that attempt. I threw out another feeble blow, saying, "But I get migraines. Any kind of stress on my neck and I'll get a migraine."

Another smile. "Not to worry. You can take your Imitrex without any problem."

In the end, we decided to wait another six weeks. There was still no actual hole in the macula, and thus still a slight chance this nightmare might end without intervention.

I started reading up on face-down recovery. Most of the information on the internet was provided by vitrectomy equipment rental companies, but still it was helpful and informative. The equipment didn't look too gruesome. It was basically repurposed massage equipment. How bad could something be if it involved massage equipment?

* * *

Time passed and the next appointment rolled around. I knew my vision had not improved. But, I had been wrong about the state of my sight before the previous visit. Maybe I was wrong this time as well. Maybe it had really gotten better unbeknownst to me. That is how I conned myself into setting foot into the retinologist's office for what I sensed would be essentially a pre-op visit.

My first clue that surgery was imminent was that the doctor entered the exam room brandishing several glossy pamphlets. He'd never done that before. Sure enough, they contained information about vitrectomy, macular hole, and face-down recovery equipment rental.

My OCT told the grim truth: two small holes had formed in my macula. And, the vitreous was still clinging to the retina like a stubborn shipping label to a worn cardboard box. Vitrectomy was in order.

I almost felt relieved. At least I wouldn't have to undergo injections into my eye, although a couple of friends had assured me the injections they'd had in their eyes had been hardly noticeable. I pictured myself blithely chattering away while the doctor stuck a needle into my eye. The image shattered when I began to imagine the needle bending as I struggled and screamed. Plus, I remembered a little incident where a friend had started saying how the eye injections *she'd* had were incredibly painful. At least, I think that's what she had been going to say. She never did finish her sentence because another friend changed the subject with lightening speed while a third friend pulled painful-eye-injection-friend into the kitchen to help with some sort of emergency there. I sensed a cover-up, but hadn't thought it wise to pursue the topic. Injections: for me, not so much.

So, great. I wasn't going to be having intraocular injections. I was going to be having a vitrectomy. Yee-ha!

"Look," I said, leaning forward in the exam chair. "Eyes gross me out. I worked in the operating room for most of my adult life and eye cases just aren't something I can stomach. When I worked in the OR, if I was assigned to a fifteen-minute eye case, I would trade it for a twelve-hour craniotomy just so I wouldn't have to look at someone cutting into an eyeball. I do not want to know anything about what you are doing with my eye."

The doctor said, "So, a general, then," and made a mark on a slip of yellow paper attached to a clipboard near the sink in the dimly lit exam room.

I relaxed a bit. I had thought I might have to argue my case for a general anesthetic a little more forcefully, but this had been easy.

"Now, about blocking the optic nerve." I held my right thumb and forefinger as far apart as they would go—about six inches—and gestured toward my right eye.

"I usually do a block for pain control," he said.

"Good thinking," I replied. Pain control: I would take as much of that as I could get.

He explained that he would put in the block after I was asleep. I was ecstatic. Further description of the surgical procedure was met with, "I don't care what you do. I'll be asleep. You just do anything you want once I'm out."

So, a decision had been made. I would have surgery in just a few weeks.

2

The Secret is in Good Preparation.

Oddly enough, I was able to keep fairly calm in the days and weeks leading up to the surgery. My mantra became, "I'll be asleep. I won't know anything about what they're doing."

I occupied my time with research into face-down recovery. What follows is the information I gleaned from a couple of books and beau coups of web pages, pamphlets, blogs, and equipment-rental sites.

Mainly, I learned that preparation is of paramount importance. It will not be any fun at all to set up or even adjust equipment after surgery. The operative day is not the time to learn that you cannot see the toilet paper in the master bathroom. I decided to make a list of preparations I felt would be most helpful to me.

Early (2-3 Weeks) Pre-op Prep

Equipment: I checked out several different suppliers. There were tons of rental places on the internet, plus my doctor gave me some brochures of rental establishments he was aware of. A couple of places gave a discount to patients of my doctor. Keep in mind that your doctor may well ask you to wear either glasses or a metal or plastic eye protector at all times during the face-down recovery period. I wore *both* for the first three days. So, carefully check out the face cradle pads made to adjust for eye glasses—you will most probably need to use this feature. Once you've made your choice, go on and reserve your equipment. You don't want to be ordering equipment the day before your procedure. I ordered mine several weeks prior to my surgery.

House: I did a preliminary tour of my house, thinking how it would be to do my daily activities while in a face-down posture.

Bathroom: I realized I would need to move toothpaste and dental floss from the medicine cabinet to the counter. Wash-clothes and towels would also need to be moved from high shelves to something lower or to the counter. I looked at the toilet paper and realized I probably would not be able to see it while my right eye was patched. I made a mental note to get a box or something on which to put toilet paper temporarily.

Closet: I would need blouses that buttoned up the front—I certainly didn't want to injure my eye while donning a pullover tee-shirt. I inventoried my supply of button-up blouses and made plans to launder and set aside those I would wear post-op. I did the same for easy-to-put-on and comfortable slacks. Then, I planned how to clear space on the lower clothes rack to accommodate the outfits I had chosen. I also looked at my shoe rack with an eye to rearranging it so I could easily reach the shoes I would likely wear while face-down.

Bedroom: I could not imagine me, a bulky face-down sleeping apparatus, my husband, and our dog all in one queen sized bed. But, I did not know what to do about it at this point. I made a mental note to figure something out.

My underwear was already in a perfect place for easy reach while face-down, so I checked that off my list.

Kitchen: I could see the coffee maker while face-down, but I would need to move sweetener packets to the counter from the cabinet where I normally kept them. The toaster would have to stay on the counter instead of being tucked away down below as normal. The refrigerator would need some major rearranging in order to put my most-used items within sight of a face-down self. It needed to be cleaned anyway, so I put off rearranging until then. I tried eating in various positions at the table and using a bar stool rather than my regular kitchen chair. Nothing seemed comfortable, but the bar stool seemed most promising. More on this later.

Family Room: I scouted out a couple of places to put the vitrectomy chair. I planned to move it from the dining room in the morning to the family room for the afternoon and on to the TV room for the evening. Little did I know that it wouldn't matter much where the chair was placed.

Week Before Surgery

Laundry: I washed the clothes I would wear after surgery. I also washed sheets, blankets, and enough towels/washcloths so that I would have a clean set each morning. I had noted that the rental company said it would be helpful to put a sheet or beach towel over the rented sleep pad, so I made sure I had something clean for that.

Vitrectomy Notebook: Aside from the file folder where I kept all the paperwork pertaining to the surgery, I began a notebook with information my husband would need to care for me, our little dog, and the house while I was face-down.

Equipment: I had the idea to use a massage table we already owned for sleeping instead of the sleep equipment I would rent. I checked this out and found it fairly comfortable. Using the massage table would also take care of the problem of our crowded bed. Furthermore, the doctor had instructed me not to allow pets in my bed during the post-op period. The massage table would solve that problem as well.

Dog: Our dog takes daily medication. I made sure I had a plastic pill organizer big enough to hold all her meds for the two weeks following my surgery. I also made arrangements with our neighbor to care for the dog on the day of my operation.

Support: My husband works from home, so we knew he would be nearby during my recovery. He cleared his calendar, though, for the two weeks following my surgery so he would be able to care for me, our dog, and the house. Neighbors and my church family planned meals to be brought in for us the entire week after surgery. This proved to be immensely helpful.

I thought my husband would almost certainly have to go out to get prescriptions filled for me immediately after surgery, so we made arrangements with a neighbor to sit with me while he was out of the house.

Shopping: I bought enough tissue boxes to place anywhere I thought I might sit or lie down after the surgery. I had read that excessive tearing might create a need for lots of tissues.

I also made sure I had enough staples (sweetener packets for coffee, butter, cream cheese, bagels, etc) in the house to last the entire face-down period.

Hair Care: I have long hair and I didn't want it trailing into my eyes after surgery. So, I made arrangements with my hairdresser to braid my hair the morning of my surgery, which luckily was scheduled for the afternoon. I also bought some crocheted hairnet/cap things and some headbands with Velcro closures. I later found a banana-type hair clip to be of great use, so I would recommend buying one of those as well if you don't already have one. I used mine to keep myself from rolling over onto my back while sleeping.

Glasses: I got a string-type eyeglass securer on the internet. I didn't want my eyeglasses slipping down my nose while I was face-down.

Food: I made it known to neighbors, friends, and my church family that I would welcome any and all meals as I wouldn't be able to cook during the recovery period.

After I had done all that, I started cleaning. We have a cleaning service, but I still cleaned my house from top to bottom. It kept my mind off the upcoming surgery.

Last Two Days Before Surgery

Closet: I got out an old shower stool, cleaned it thoroughly, and set it in my closet as an easy-visibility holder for towels and wash clothes. I put all the clothes I wanted to wear post-op on a lower rack and moved appropriate shoes to lower positions in the shoe rack.

Bathroom: I made sure my new Velcro headbands and crocheted hairnets were in a lower drawer, along with my hairbrush, tooth-brush, etc. I moved the toothpaste and dental floss from the medicine cabinet to the counter. I put my suction-type soap holder at a lower position in the shower so I would be able to see it easily. I also put some boxes on the left side of each toilet and placed a roll of toilet paper on each of them so that I could see the toilet paper while blind in my right eye.

Shopping: I bought a bunch of treats, cookies and such, that I thought would cheer me up while doing my time face-down. I also bought some alcohol swabs (for cleaning the metal eye protector) and some cotton rounds that I thought I might use in the eye area. I didn't want to use plain cotton balls for wiping around my eye as I had an idea they might catch on my eyelashes and leave wisps of cotton there, which I knew would drive me crazy.

Equipment: My husband and I set up the rental equipment and got it adjusted to fit my body. I had decided to use a massage table, which we already had, to sleep on rather than the sleep thing we had rented. So, I set the massage table up in the bedroom and set up the rented sleep equipment in the guest bedroom for naps or in case the massage table proved to be not as comfortable as I hoped. I found a thing called a Float on the internet and purchased one. The Float is a device that fits between the face cradle frame and the face pads (either the three-pad adjustable set or the horseshoe-shaped pad.) It allows for some motion of the head and neck while using the face cradle. I found it very helpful—in fact, I couldn't sleep without it—but a friend who also underwent face-down recovery found the Float very uncomfortable and never used it.

I also tried out my Kindle **with** the seating equipment. Placing the face rest at a height comfortable for my neck put the Kindle at an impossible distance for reading. So, I knew I needed to download some audible books to keep me entertained during the face-down period.

Entertainment/Distraction Options: I knew keeping myself distracted and entertained would be a crucial part of maintaining a face-down position for an entire week or more. Having realized that reading, either regular books or my Kindle, would not be convenient because of my prospective seating arrangement, I considered audible books the next best thing. I downloaded some from both my public library and from Amazon. Then, I tried out at least one from each source just make sure I could actually use them on my device. Only after doing this did I begin to search for the books I would enjoy during my recovery period. When I found some, I downloaded them and made sure they worked properly. I also downloaded and tested a couple of movies and a few TV dramas. Luckily I had the foresight to place a stylus for the Kindle screen at each place where I would use the Kindle. This proved very helpful as for some reason it was troublesome to use my fingers to manipulate the Kindle post-op.

This next part seems silly, but it truly helped me after the surgery. I found several photos that I liked and mounted them on thick paper, then covered them with plastic wrap. I placed these on all the surfaces that would be visible to me as I sat in my rental equipment. It certainly beat staring down at blank surfaces when I was visiting with friends or just too tired to concentrate on videos or audio books.

Kitchen: I cleaned out the refrigerator only because it really needed it. (If it hadn't been so filthy, I would have merely done some rearrangement.) When I replaced the food, I made sure to put items I thought I would want to reach for myself on lower shelves. I placed sweetener for coffee in a lower cabinet. I put cookies and treats on the counter where I could grab them at will. The toaster went on the counter and would remain there within easy reach until I was upright again. Mainly, I just put needed items where I would be able to see them without raising my head.

Bedroom: For maximum sleeping comfort, I placed an egg-crate mattress pad on top of the massage table. I put linens over that and adjusted the face cradle, with the Float in place so that my neck was in good alignment. I also placed a box of tissues and several small pillows within easy reach of the massage table. I wish I had thought to place a washcloth or paper towel on the shelf below the face cradle. It turned out that I drooled a lot while sleeping face down. A cloth below my face would have been convenient.

Self: The hospital provided anti-bacterial soap for me to use in the days prior to my surgery. I washed with it religiously as instructed. I also made sure to drink plenty of fluids and get lots of sleep in the last few days before my operation. And, I washed my hair the morning of surgery before having it braided by my hair dresser. I figured it would be a while until I could shampoo it again.

Car: I placed the rented travel block in the backseat of the car while my husband made sure the area where I would sit was clear of debris. (We keep a bit of dog equipment in the backseat of our car as the dog often goes with us on short journeys. Some of this needed to be moved to the trunk of the car.)

3

Surgery Day

I woke up early on the day of my surgery despite my best efforts to sleep in. Before going to bed, I had placed notes on both the coffee pot and the toaster to remind myself of the requirement to go without food or fluids until after the surgery.

I met my hairdresser at her shop and had my hair braided. She included my bangs in the braid to insure that no stray hairs would trail down into my eye.

By the time I arrived at home, it was time to leave for the hospital. The fact that I nearly ran over my husband because I did not see him waving his arms as I pulled into the driveway made me realize how much my vision had deteriorated. The poor guy actually had to jump out of the way of my car! After that scary incident, I knew surgery was the right thing to do. I really probably should not have been driving, but that is a topic for another book.

We arrived at the hospital in good time and found an excellent parking place. A couple from our church met us in the waiting area and the adventure began.

Very soon after finding a cozy spot in the waiting room, I was summoned by the pre-op nurse. We went to a small room where I replaced my clothing with a hospital gown and plastic id bracelet. After some preliminary questions, the nurse got my IV started and asked if I wanted to see my husband and friends. I said I would like that.

With Gary and my friend in the room, I got several doses of eye drops and talked with the anesthesiologist who would be in charge of my case. The pre-op nurse had me identify which eye we would be working on and placed a rub-on tattoo over that eye. Eventually, my surgeon dropped in and placed his initials near that tattoo to indicate that he agreed that was the correct eye. All this reassured me immensely.

Next, I got some pre-op medication through my IV and don't remember much more although my husband says I carried on a sort of drunken conversation with him right up to the time I was wheeled off to the operating room.

During the operation, my husband sat in the waiting room where he was supported by conversation with our friends from church. The presence of friendly faces during our time at the hospital was very helpful, both to him and to me.

The next thing I knew, I was sitting up in a stretcher sipping Sprite. I said I didn't think I was allowed to have fluids before surgery and the nurse told me the operation was over. "Oh," I said. My friend and my husband helped me put my clothes on and the nurse wheeled me out to the car.

I sat in the back passenger seat because I had read somewhere that this is the safest position in a car. In case of a minor traffic accident, I did not want the airbag going off and injuring my newly-operated eye. My husband handed me the travel block as soon as I had buckled my seatbelt and we headed for home.

I could barely see. The face cradle limited my vision to a small area directly in front of my face. My right eye (the one they had operated on) was covered by a cotton patch with a metal eye protector securely taped over that. Plus, my good eye didn't seem to be working as well as it normally did. I was glad I had placed a photo of a cute dog on the travel block prior to putting it in the car, although I had to really concentrate to focus on it.

The car swung wildly, almost throwing me off the travel block. "What was that?" I asked. My husband explained that he had just made a very gentle left turn. I asked him to tell me before making any further turns so I could hang onto the seat in front of me for balance. This worked well on all subsequent trips with the travel block.

We arrived at home, where we were met by the neighbor who was caring for our dog and who had also agreed to babysit me while Gary went to have my prescriptions filled. I sat at the kitchen table in my special equipment and sipped some cranberry juice. My eye didn't really hurt, but it felt like it might be going to start any minute.

I took some pain medicine as well as some medicine for nausea as soon as it was available. The neighbor left and I settled in for a week of face-down recovery.

It seemed to me that lying face-down would be even less comfortable than sitting in the face-down chair, so I sat up and tried to focus on the photo I had placed nearby. It was about all I could do. Audio books, video, or even conversation seemed beyond my capability at that moment.

Soon, my husband served me a scrambled egg, two pieces of toast, and a little Jell-O. Eating exhausted me, but the thought of lying face-down just wasn't appealing. So, I sat face-down and looked at my little photo wrapped in plastic wrap until bedtime. It was amazing how difficult it was to see even though my left eye was supposedly not affected by the surgery.

Finally, it was late enough that we had to go to bed. My husband helped me to the bathroom where I wiped my face with a damp wash-cloth and brushed my teeth. After a final dose of pain and nausea medicine, I climbed onto the torture rack massage table with quite a bit of assistance from my husband. It took a seemingly endless amount of time to get the face pads adjusted to a tolerable degree of comfort. With the bulky eye dressing in place, it seemed there was no way to support my head without excessive pressure on the rim of the metal eye protector. Plus, the pads pulled at my skin in a particularly maddening way. After what seemed like just a few minutes, my face would slide through the pads until I was hanging by my ears and I would have to readjust once more. This awful sequence repeated throughout the night. I felt around and found a couple of the small pillows I had placed near my bed prior to leaving for the hospital. I jammed one pillow under each shoulder. It helped a little. My discharge instructions said I was allowed to sleep on either side or face-down, but I wanted to stay face-down as much as possible to insure the very best outcome. So, I spent a very uncomfortable night lying face down, drooling when I did manage to doze off, and rearranging the face-pads every little while.

My poor, dear husband fared no better. He woke up every time I moved. The face pads were attached with Velcro so every time I pulled them off to try and get comfortable, it sounded like Godzilla was ripping the roof off our house.

4

Face-Down Recovery

The next morning, I had an appointment with my surgeon in Greenville. So, we loaded up and drove over there with me using my travel block and clutching the seat in front of me during turns and curves.

Gary, toting the bulky travel block, guided me into the office. I rested my head on the face pads while I waited. It didn't matter where I was: my world consisted of the one square foot in front of my downturned face. Soon, a disembodied voice called my name. I raised my hand and the caller offered me her arm for guidance to the exam room.

Once safely deposited with the tech who would conduct my preliminary exams, I sat with my face up for the first time since the operation. The tech removed my eye dressings and asked if I could identify the letters on the vision chart she claimed was in front of me. I couldn't even see the chart, much less read anything written on it. All I saw was a kind of blank whiteness dissected by a jagged black line that shimmered sickeningly. A shadow appeared in front of me. "Can you see me?" a voice asked.

"Uh, there's a shadow that might be you," I said.

"Can you see how many fingers I'm holding up?"

A pair of pinkish dots swam close to my face. "Two?" I asked, not really sure what I was seeing.

The voice assured me that my lack of vision was normal the day after surgery.

Eventually, I was led to another chair and my doctor's voice warned me of an impending exam with the slit lamp.

* * *

I am allergic to most kinds of tape. I can tolerate paper tape fairly well, but the less skin/tape contact, the better for me. After the slit-lamp exam, my doctor said I could dispense with the eye patch/protector and just wear my glasses, but the bizarre visual distortion in my right eye bothered me so much that I wanted to keep that eye covered. I tried just closing the right eye, but that got very tiring very quickly. We ended up placing an eye pad over the metal eye protector and holding the whole thing in place with my glasses, which were well-secured by the elastic holder-thingie I had purchased before surgery.

The bothersome distortion lasted about three days, after which I was able to tolerate wearing only my glasses during the day. I taped the eye protector in place at night, however, until I saw the doctor for my one-week post-op visit and got his permission to do without it at night.

I really had almost no eye pain during the entire week of face-down recovery. My neck, back, and hips were another matter, however. I found I could not tolerate more than about forty five minutes of sitting in the rental chair without having to get up and walk around a little.

After two days, I decided that the rental equipment was supposed to be an aid to my comfort, not a prison. My face was getting sore and feeling raw from taping the eye protector on at night as well as from constantly rubbing against the face pads of the vitrectomy support equipment. I got creative and used every chest pad they had sent. Instead of resting my arms on the support in front of the chair, I often put them on the chest pad. I tried every position I could concoct, just to change things up. Still, my neck, shoulders, and back ached by the end of each day. Looking back, I would take more pain medicine for those aches if I had it to do over again.

Every day, I made it a point to walk outside a little bit with my husband's help. At first, I barely made it to the mailbox at the end of our driveway. By the end of the week, I was able to walk to the neighbor's driveway entrance without becoming over-tired.

Nights were a problem. I just couldn't sleep much in the face-down position. I tend to move around a lot during the night anyway and remaining in one position was virtually impossible for me. By the third night, I decided to follow my doctor's instructions and slept at least part of each night on my side. That helped immensely. It also gave the skin on my face some relief from the constant pulling and pressure of the face pads.

Neighbors and church family provided meals for us throughout the week. It was a godsend. I don't think we could have coped if my husband had been obliged to prepare meals as well as take care of me, the house, and our dog.

Eating face-down was not pretty. I ended up sitting at our kitchen bar on a bar stool with a plate of food in my lap. I would lean my head against the table seating support between bites. Things went easier if I held the plate close to my mouth and kind of scooped food in. Not a process I wanted anyone to see! Our little dog soon learned that the area around my chair was a rich source of dropped food, though, so at least one family member profited from my awkward meals.

Eventually, I felt more alert, although still uncomfortable from staying in a face-down position. The solution for me was to move around as much as possible without compromising the face-down positioning. I spent a lot of time pacing around the house. Every hour or so, I would rest my head on a counter or the back of a couch and stretch my legs, back and neck as much as possible.

Toward the end of the recovery period, I even did some laundry—sort of. My husband would bring baskets of dirty clothes and set them on the dryer for me. I would sort them and dump a load into the washer, then toss a load into the dryer after the wash cycle finished. Finally, Gary would carry the clean laundry into the dining room, where I would fold it and put away as much as I could. Doing this made me feel I was contributing to the household work and decreased my back and neck pain as well.

I also made my own breakfast, which consisted of a toasted bagel, some blueberries, cream cheese, coffee, and a soft drink of some kind. It was very empowering to be able to go into the kitchen and prepare this for myself.

I bathed every night except the very first—the night of my surgery. This was not easy, but it relaxed me and made me feel ready for bed. Gary would help me into the tub, wash my back for me, then wait nearby until I called for help getting out of the tub. I ran a clean, damp wash-cloth over my face before getting into the bath so as to avoid washing my face with water in which I was sitting. I wore my glasses in the tub to protect my eye from injury.

About the middle of the week, my hair felt filthy to me. So, I checked with my surgeon to make sure a shampoo would be okay. With his blessing, I showered and washed my hair, being careful not to get any water or soap into my eye. Gary stood just outside the shower and provided a clean, dry face towel as needed during the procedure. I even dried my hair with a blow dryer afterwards. From that time on, I held my hair back with a banana clip and kept my bangs under control with one of the Velcro-fastened headbands I had purchased before going to the hospital.

The banana clip came in very handy for more than simply keeping my long hair under control. I had read that some vitrectomy patients tape a tennis ball to their back at bedtime in order to prevent them from rolling over onto their back while sleeping. That was out for me due to my tape allergy. I had bought some bras to sleep in and had devised a system involving a safety pin, a sock, and a dryer ball to accomplish the same purpose as taping a tennis ball onto my back. But, Gary very kindly gave me a back massage every night before sleep. The bra system interfered with that. After my shampoo and subsequent use of the banana clip for hair control, I realized that there was no way I could sleep face-up with one of those things (the banana clip) on the back of my head. So, I just left a banana clip in place when I lay down to sleep and worried no more about rolling over onto my back without waking up.

Just when I was on the point of trying to find some kind of protective cream for the skin on my face—the nightly taping and daily pulling and pressure of the face pads was really causing problems for me—it was time for my one-week post-op visit with my surgeon. I did the eye-chart vision exam and could read an amazing number of lines. The doctor gave me permission to be face-up during the day and to sleep on either side or face-down. My face-down recovery period was finished!!

5

Here is a summary of the things I found helpful.

1. Good preparation. Having the house and equipment ready when I came home from the hospital was a no-brainer.

2. Community support. They say it takes a village to raise a child, and I say it takes a village to recover a vitrectomy patient. We absolutely could not have done it without help from our friends, neighbors, and church family.

3. Frequent change of position. I could not have recovered without moving around as much as possible within the confines of the prescribed posture.

4. Hair control. It would have driven me insane to have hair hanging down into my eyes during the face-down period.

5. Pre-downloaded audio books. These kept me entertained with almost no effort on my part. Videos were okay, but I found them a little tiring to watch. Watching TV through the mirror exhausted me.

6. Banana clip in the hair to prevent rolling over onto the back while sleeping. A simple solution to a big worry.

7. A nightly back and foot rub from my husband was the best part of every day. I might even go so far as to say it was the *only*

good part of some days!

6

And, some things that didn't work as well as planned.

1. The whole dryer ball in a sock pinned to a sleep bra idea. Just put a banana clip in the hair and you're done.

2. My husband had envisioned a lot of time to work on the computer while sitting calmly by my side. It turned out he was constantly busy and had almost no time for anything but caring for me, the house, and the dog. And that was with meals being delivered daily!

3. The equipment being totally all you need for comfort. It was comfortable, but I couldn't just sit quietly for hours on end. I had to get creative, sit all kinds of ways, and walk around just to maintain a modicum of comfort while face-down.

4. TV watching. I had planned to watch lots of TV using the mirror from the equipment rental company. While I could certainly see the TV just fine using the mirror, I couldn't seem to sit still long enough to watch an entire show that way. Kindle video was better, but still required more concentration than I could muster most days.

5. Resting my head on the face pads. Don't get me wrong, I could not have endured face-down recovery without the rented

vitrectomy equipment. But, it was not the be-all and end-all of positioning. I needed quite a bit of time with my face not in contact with anything. That meant devising ways to support my head against the wall, placing just my forehead on a horseshoe cushion on the table in front of me, walking around with my face down, etc.

7

Conclusion

I hope the story of my experience with vitreomacular traction, vitrectomy, and face-down recovery has helped in some small way.

Remember to follow your own doctor's instructions rather than relying on anything in this book as this is simply one person's story rather than a medical guide.

II

Checklists

These are checklists I used to get ready for my vitrectomy surgery. They were an aid to preparation for the big day. More importantly, though, they helped me keep busy instead of sitting and worrying!

8

One or Two Weeks Before Surgery

Kitchen:

- Necessary foods, appliances accessible or have a plan to make them easy to reach
- Do a trial run of eating while in face-down position
- Obtain straws and lidded cups for post-op use

Bathroom:

- Toilet paper on side of "good" eye or have a plan to put it where it can be seen post-op
- Toiletries accessible or plan to make them so

Closet:

- Check for clothing that will need to be laundered
- No pull-over tops
- Plan a place to put clothing for ease of use post-op

- Shoes accessible or have a plan to make them so

Bedroom:

- Sleeping arrangement planned out
- Plan a convenient place for: small pillows, audio book device if you want one, tissues.

Day Room:

- Scout out a place for the post-op chair
- Make sure the TV will be visible from the chair through use of the mirror
- Make sure any devices you will use during post-op period are in working order. This might include Kindle or other e-reader, tablet device, TV, radio, music player.

Self check:

- Any hair problems that might drive you crazy while face-down? Make plans to deal with problems you identify.
- Any grooming procedures you want done prior to going in for surgery? These might include nail polish removal, shampoo, or a good shave. Make appointments if necessary or plan time to do this sort of thing yourself before you leave for surgery.

Support Systems:

- Arrange for someone to drive you home from the hospital after surgery
- Arrange for someone to watch dog, house, etc during surgery
- Have someone to assist you during face-down period
- Let it be known that you will welcome meals after surgery
- Consider having someone accompany you and your primary support person to the hospital on the day of surgery
- Set up a vitrectomy notebook: include anything those caring for you might need to know. For instance pet's schedule, plant watering schedule, how to run the washing machine, when the cleaning service comes and how they are paid. Consider adding a blank page to jot down things like food people bring, flowers sent by friends, addresses for thank you notes

If you plan to rent vitrectomy equipment

- Check out various sources for equipment
- Decide what equipment you want to rent
- Arrange to have the equipment delivered two or three days before your surgery so you can set it up at a leisurely pace

9

Two or Three Days Before Surgery

Bathroom

- Put toilet paper where you will be able to see it post-op
- Place toiletries on counter or in easily-reached drawer
- Have towels and wash-clothes on a low shelf or bench

Closet

- Have easy-to-put-on clothing ready for day of surgery
- Have post-op clothes clean and accessible
- Place shoes where you can put them on easily

Bedroom

- Set up sleeping items (may need to be done right before leaving for hospital, depending on your planned method)

- Clean linens on sleeping area
- Tissues available
- Small pillows nearby

Kitchen

- Rearrange refrigerator for ease of use post-op
- Put food items and small appliances where they can be used while face-down
- Meal-time accommodations in place (rented table-seat, bar stool, etc)
- Straws and lidded cups in an easy-to-reach place
- Some provision for post-op meals, whether having food brought in or just a number of casseroles in the freezer
- Special foods prepared and available, such as gelatin desserts, juice or other drink, easy-to-eat snacks.

Day room

- Vitrectomy chair set up, adjusted for comfort, and in place
- Tissues easily available
- Some accommodation for used tissues/other trash. A plastic bag taped near the vitrectomy chair works well.

Entertainment Options

- E-reader/tablet in working order
- Preferred content downloaded and ready to play

- Plug and charge cord conveniently located
- Mirror adjusted properly
- TV where it can be seen through mirror
- Support
- Reading material/e-entertainment ready for waiting room use by primary support person

Support Group

- Arrangements made for communicating with distant family and friends post-op, if needed
- You may want someone to notify far-away family/friends of your progress

Car

- Have someone available to drive you home after surgery
- Have travel block in place for trip home from hospital
- Make sure you have adequate fuel in car for: trip to and from the hospital, trip to pharmacy to fill post-op prescriptions, post-op visits to the surgeon's office.
- Make sure driver (spouse, friend, etc) has directions to hospital and knows the correct entrance for surgery patients. The driver will also need to know how to get to the surgeon's office for your post visits.

If you rent equipment

- Confirm delivery
- Set up equipment when available
- Adjust equipment as needed
- Practice using equipment. Make sure you can get in and out of the chair without difficulty. Try sipping from a straw while using the head cradle attached to the dining table.

10

Shopping List

- Pantry Staples (i.e. bread, milk, cereal, etc)
- Easy-to-eat treats
- Juices, soft drinks for post-op enjoyment
- Gelatin dessert mix if you think you might want it post-op
- Hair Care
- Crocheted hair nets
- Velcro headbands
- Banana Clip NOT JUST FOR HAIR—KEEPS YOU FROM ROLLING ONTO YOUR BACK WHILE SLEEPING
- Tissues to place near every chair and the bed
- Audio books
- Videos
- Egg crate mattress pad, if desired
- Float for between face pad and face cradle frame, if desired. I ordered my Boiance Float online from Oakworks http://www.massagetables.com/boiance-float.aspx
- Lotion for back and foot massages
- Alcohol wipes—good for cleaning small items
- Cotton rounds—I used them for gentle cleaning near the eye
- Tape to secure eye protector, also can be used to tape trash bags for used tissues near seating

- Disinfectant wipes—we used them for quick kitchen clean-up
- Easy-to-put-on clothing, if not already available
- Several small containers of hand sanitizer. I kept them near each chair I sat in and used them to clean my hands after petting the dog.
- String-type holder to keep eyeglasses in place while face-down
- Rental vitrectomy equipment, if desired

Made in the USA
Monee, IL
09 May 2021